PREFACE.

In issuing this little book I have been actuated by a desire to do something towards the removal of a lamentable degree of popular ignorance.

It seems that no proposition that can be made is so absurd or impossible but that many people, ordinarily regarded as intelligent, will be found to accept it and to aid in its propagation. And hence, when it is asserted that a young lady has lived for fourteen years without food of any kind, hundreds and thousands of persons throughout the length and breadth of a civilized land at once yield their belief to the monstrous declaration.

I have confined my remarks entirely to the question of abstinence from food. The other supernatural gifts, the possession of which is claimed, would, if considered, have extended the limits of this little volume beyond the bounds which were deemed expedient. At some future time I may be tempted to discuss them. In the meantime it is well to call to mind that a proposition (*see* Appendix) which I made solely in the interest of truth was disregarded, ostensibly with the desire to avoid publicity, when in fact the daily press had for weeks been filled with reports in detail, furnished by the friends of the young lady in question, of the marvellous powers she was said to possess.

A portion of this essay, which bore upon the matter discussed, has been taken from another volume by the author, published several years ago, and now out of print.

WILLIAM A. HAMMOND.

CONTENTS

		PAGE
I	Abstinence in the Middle Ages	1
II	Abstinence in Modern Times	6
III	Abstinence from Food, with Stigmatization	31
IV	The Brooklyn Case	48
V	The Physiology and Pathology of Inanition	59

FASTING GIRLS.

I.

ABSTINENCE IN THE MIDDLE AGES.

Among the many remarkable manifestations by which hysteria exhibits itself, for the astonishment of the credulous and uneducated portion of the public, and—alas, that it should have to be said,—for the delectation of an occasional weak-minded and ignorant physician, the assumption of the ability to live without food may be assigned a prominent place. I am not aware that this power has been claimed in its fullest development for the male of the human species. When he is deprived of food he dies in a few days, more or less, according to his physical condition as regards adipose tissue and strength of constitution; but if a weak emaciated girl asserts that she is able to exist for years without eating, there are at once certificates and letters from clergymen, professors, and even physicians, in support of the truth of her story. The element of impossibility goes for nothing against the bare word of such a woman, and her statements are accepted with a degree of confidence which is lamentable to witness in this era of the world's progress.

The class of deceptions occasionally induced by hysteria, and embracing these "fasting girls," has been known for many years, though it is only in comparatively recent times that the instances have been taken at their proper value. Görres[1] gives a number of examples occurring among male and female saints and other holy persons, in which partial or total abstinence from food was said to have existed for long periods.

Thus Liduine of Schiedam fell ill in 1395, and remained in that state till her death, thirty-three years subsequently. During the first nineteen years she ate every day nothing but a little piece of apple the size of a holy wafer, and drank a little water and a swallow of beer, or sometimes a little sweet milk. Subsequently, being unable to digest beer and milk, she restricted herself to a little wine and water, and still later she was obliged to confine herself to water alone, which served her both as food and drink. But after nineteen years she took nothing whatever, according to her own statement made to some friars in 1422, she averring that for eight years nothing in the way of nourishment had passed her lips, and that for twenty years she had seen neither the sun nor the moon, nor had touched the earth with her feet.

Saint Joseph of Copertino remained for five years without eating bread, and ten years without drinking wine, contenting himself with dried fruits, which he mixed with various bitter herbs. The herb which he used for Fridays had such an atrocious taste, that one of the brethren, by simply putting his tongue to it, was seized with vomiting, and for several days thereafter everything he ate excited nausea. He fasted for forty days seven times every year, and during these periods ate nothing at all except on Sundays and Thursdays.

Nicolas of Flue, as soon as he embraced the monastic life, subsisted altogether on the holy eucharist. The pious Görres in explanation of this miracle says:

"In ordinary nourishment he who eats being superior to that which is eaten, assimilates the aliments which he takes, and communicates to them his own nature. But in the eucharist the aliment is more powerful than he who eats. It is no longer therefore the nourishment which is assimilated, but on the contrary, it assimilates the man, and introduces him into a superior sphere. An entire change is produced. The supernatural life in some way or other absorbs the natural life, and the man instead of living on earth, lives henceforth by grace and by heaven."

This is about on a par, as regards lucidity and logic, with the explanations which we are given of the alleged case of prolonged fasting in Brooklyn.

Doubts arose in regard to Nicolas, and the bishop had him watched, but without detecting him in fraud. Finally he ordered him to eat a piece of bread in his presence. Nicolas did as he was commanded, but at the first mouthful he was seized with violent vomiting. The bishop inquired of him how he thus managed to live without eating, to which the brother answered that when he assisted at mass, and when he took the holy eucharist, he felt a degree of strength and suppleness like that derived from the most nutritious food.

Still the doubters continued, and the inhabitants of Underwold, where Nicolas lived, appear to have been at first very much inclined to suspect him of deceit. But they were finally converted, for having during a whole month guarded every approach to his cabin, and having during that time detected no one in taking food to him, they were convinced that for that time at least he had lived without food. The sceptical reasoner of the present day would probably regard the test as insufficient.

In 1225, Hugh, Bishop of Lincoln, having heard that there was at Leicester a nun who had taken no nourishment for seven years, and who lived only on the eucharist, which she took every Sunday, gave at first no faith to the story. He sent to her, however, fifteen clerks, with directions to watch her assiduously for fifteen days, never for an instant losing sight of her. The clerks reported to him that they had strictly obeyed his commands; that she had taken no nourishment, and that yet she nevertheless preserved her full strength and health. Whereupon the Bishop declared himself convinced, "as," adds Görres, "it was proper for a sensible man to do."

Among others of the holy persons who acquired the power of living on the sacramental bread, may be mentioned St. Catharine of Sienna, Saint Rose of Lima, Saint Collete, Saint Peter of Alcantara, and many others.

But if saints and other holy people were able, through miraculous power, to live without food, the same ability was claimed for those who were under the influence of demons and devils. Görres[2] states that a person possessed by a devil often loses all taste for food of any kind, and can retain no nourishment in his body. Another symptom is a disgust which is formed for the companionship of other persons. Thus a man was tormented by a demon, who forced him to fly into the forests, where he hid himself from mankind. One night he quit his house, and concealed himself in a cavern, remaining there entirely without food for sixteen days. Again he remained in the woods twenty-four days, neither eating nor drinking during this period. Finally his children found him, and taking him to a priest, had the devil exorcised, and he was cured.

Saint Prosper, of Aquitaine, speaks of a young girl possessed by a devil, and who went seventy days without eating. Notwithstanding this long fast, she did not become emaciated, because every night at twelve o'clock a bird sent by the devil took a mysterious nourishment to her.

An astonishing feature in the cases of the diabolical abstaining from food, is that, as in the holy instances, they exhibit various manifestations of hysteria. Görres, with a charming degree of simplicity, details these symptoms and failing, under the influence of the predominant idea which fills him, to recognize their real character, ascribes them without hesitation to devilish agency. Thus he says:

"The functions of the organs of nutrition are sometimes profoundly altered in the possessed, and these alterations are manifested by violent cramps, which show the extent to which the muscular system is affected. The hysterical lump in the throat is a frequent phenomenon in possession. A young girl in the Valley of Calepino had all her limbs twisted and contracted, and had in the œsophagus a sensation as if a ball was sometimes rising in her throat, and again falling to her stomach. Her countenance was of an ashen hue, and she had a constant sense of weight and pain in the head. All the remedies of physicians had failed, and as evidences of possession were discovered in her, she was brought to Brignoli (a priest) who had recourse to supernatural means, and cured her."

Strange to say, the ability to live on the eucharist, and to resist starvation by diabolical power, died out with the middle ages, and was replaced by the "fasting girls," who still continue to amuse us with their vagaries. To the consideration of some of the more striking instances of more recent times the attention of the reader is invited, in the confidence that much of interest in the study of the "History of Human Folly" will be adduced.

FOOTNOTES:

[1] La Mystique Divine, Naturelle et Diabolique. Paris, 1861. t. I., p. 194, *et seq.*

[2] Op. cit. t. IV., p. 446.

II.

ABSTINENCE IN MODERN TIMES.

Among the more striking cases under this head, is that of Margaret Weiss, a young girl ten years of age, who lived at Rode, a small village near Spires, and whose history has come down to us through various channels, but principally from Gerardus Bucoldianus,[3] who had the medical charge of her, and who wrote a little book describing his patient. Margaret is said to have abstained from all food and drink for three years, in the meantime growing, walking about, laughing, and talking like other children of her age. During the first year, however, she suffered greatly from pains in her head and abdomen, and, a common condition in hysteria—all four of her limbs were contracted. She passed neither urine nor fæces. Margaret, though only ten years old—hysteria develops the secretive faculties—played her part so well that, after being watched by the priest of the parish and Dr. Bucoldianus, she was considered free from all juggling, and was sent home to her friends by order of the King, "not," the doctor adds, "without great admiration and princely gifts." Although fully accepting the fact of Margaret's abstinence, Dr. Bucoldianus appears to have been somewhat staggered, for he asks very pertinently: "Whence comes the animal heat, since she neither eats nor drinks, and why does the body grow when nothing goes into it?"

Schenckius[4] quotes from Paulus Lentulus the "Wonderful History of the Fasting of Appolonia Schreira, a virgin in Berne." Lentulus states that he was with this maid on three occasions, and that, by order of the magistrate of Berne, she was taken to that city and a strict guard kept upon her. All kinds of means were set in operation to detect imposture if any existed, but none was discovered, and she was set at liberty as a genuine case of ability to live without food. In the first year of her fasting she scarcely slept, and in the second year never closed her eyes in sleep; and so she continued for a long while after.

Schenckius also advances the case of Katharine Binder, of the Palatinate, who was closely watched by a clergyman, a statesman, and two doctors of medicine, without the detection of fraud on her part. She was said to have taken nothing but air into her system for nine years and more, as Lentulus reported on the authority of Fabricius. This last-named physician told Lentulus of another case, that of a girl fourteen years old, who certainly had taken neither food nor drink for at least three years.

"But," says Dr. Hakewel,[5] "the strangest that I have met with of this kind, is the history of Eve Fliegen, out of Dutch translated into English, and printed at London, *anno* 1611, who, being born at Meurs, is said to have taken no kind of sustenance for the space of fourteen years together; that is, from the year of her age, twenty-two to thirty-six, and from the year of our Lord 1597 to 1611; and this we have confirmed by the testimony of the magistrates of the town of Meurs, as also by the minister who made trial of her in his house thirteen days together by all the means he could devise, but could detect no imposture." Over the picture of this maid, set in front of the Dutch copy, stand these Latin verses:

> "Meursæ hæc quam cernis decies ter, sexque peregit,
> Annos, bis septem prorsus non viscitur annis
> Nec potat, sic sola sedet, sic pallida vitam
> Ducit, et exigui se oblectat floribus horti."

Thus rendered in the English copy:

> "This maid of Meurs thirty and six years spent,
> Fourteen of which she took no nourishment;
> Thus pale and wan she sits sad and alone,
> A garden's all she loves to look upon."

Franciscus Citesius,[6] physician to the King of France and to Cardinal Richelieu, devotes a good deal of space and attention to the case of Joan Balaam, a native of the city of Constance. She was well grown, but of bad manners. About the eleventh year of her age she was attacked with a fever, and among other symptoms vomited for twenty days. Then she became speechless and so continued for twenty-four days. Then she talked, but her speech was raving and incoherent. Finally she lost all power of motion and of sensibility in the parts below the head and could not swallow. From thenceforth she could not be persuaded to take food. Six months afterwards she regained the use of her limbs, but the inability to swallow remained and she acquired a great loathing for all kinds of meat and drink. The secretions and excretions appeared to be arrested. Nevertheless she was very industrious, employing her time in running errands, sweeping the house, spinning, and such like. This maid continued thus fasting for the space of nearly three years, and then by degrees took to eating and drinking again.

Before coming to more recent cases, there is one other to which I desire to refer for the reason mainly that in it there was probably organic disease in addition to fraud and hysteria. It is cited by Fabricius[7] and by Wanley. *Anno Dom.*, 1595, a maid of about thirteen years was brought out of the dukedom of Juliers to Cologne, and there in a broad street at the sign of the White Horse exposed to the sight of as many as desired to see her. The parents of this maid affirmed that she had lived without any kind of food or drink for the space of three whole years; and this they confirmed by the testimony of divers persons, such as are worthy of credit. Fabricius observed her with great care. She was of a sad and melancholy countenance; her whole body was sufficiently fleshy except only her belly, which was compressed so as that it seemed to cleave to her back-bone. Her liver and the rest of her bowels were perceived to be hard by laying the hand on the belly. As for excrements, she voided none; and did so far abhor all kinds of food, that when one, who came to see her privately, put a little sugar in her mouth she immediately swooned away. But what was most wonderful was, that this maid walked up and down, played with other girls, danced, and did all other things that were done by girls of her age; neither had she any difficulty of breathing, speaking or crying out. Her parents declared that she had been in this condition for three years.

A great many more to the same effect might be adduced, but the foregoing are sufficient to indicate the fact that belief in the possibility of such occurrences was quite general, and that if doubt did exist in regard to their real nature, it was not so strong as not readily to be overcome by the tricks and devices of hysterical women.

In the following instances of more modern date the reader will perceive the view which is taken of them by physicians of the present day, and will doubtless discover their real nature.

About sixty-five years ago, a woman of Sudbury, in Staffordshire, England, named Ann Moore, declared that she did not eat, and a number of persons volunteered to watch her, in order to ascertain whether or not she was speaking the truth. The watch was continued for three weeks and then the watchers, as in other instances, reported that Ann Moore was a real case of abstinence from food of all kinds. The Bible was always kept open on Ann's bed. Her emaciation was so extreme that it was said her vertebral column could be felt through the abdominal walls. This sad condition was asserted to have been caused by her washing the linen of a person affected with ulcers. From that time she experienced a dislike for food, and even nausea at the sight or mention of it.

As soon as the watchers reported in favor of the genuineness of Ann's pretensions her notoriety increased, and visitors came from all parts of the country, leaving donations to the extent of two hundred and fifty pounds in the course of two years. Doubts, however, again arose, and, bold from the immunity she had experienced from the first investigation, Ann in an evil moment, for the continuance of her fraud, consented to a second watching. This committee was composed of notable persons, among them being Sir Oswald Mosley, Bart., Rev. Legh Richmond, Dr. Fox, and his son, and many other gentlemen of the country. Two of them were always in her room night and day. At the suggestion of Mr. Francis Fox, the bedstead, bedding, and the woman in it were placed on a weighing machine, and thus it was ascertained that she regularly lost weight daily. At the expiration of the ninth day of this strict watching, Dr. Fox found her evidently sinking and told her she would soon die unless she took food. After a little prevarication, the woman signed a written confession that she was an impostor, and had "occasionally taken sustenance for the last six years." She also stated that during the first watch of three weeks her daughter had contrived, when washing her face, to feed her every morning, by using towels made very wet with gravy, milk, or strong arrowroot gruel, and had also conveyed food from mouth to mouth in kissing her, which it is presumed she did very often.[8]

In a clinical lecture delivered at St. George's Hospital,[9] Dr. John W. Ogle calls attention to the simulation of fasting as a manifestation of hysteria, and relates the following amusing case:

"A girl strongly hysterical, aged twenty, in spite of all persuasion and medical treatment, refused every kind of food, or if made to eat, soon vomited the contents of the stomach. On November 6th, 1869, whilst the girl was apparently suffering in the same manner, the Queen passed the hospital on her way to open Blackfriars Bridge. She arose in bed so as to look out of the window, although up to this time declaring that every movement of her body caused intense pain. On December 29, the following letter in the girl's handwriting, addressed to another patient in the same ward, was picked up from the floor: 'My Dear Mrs. Evens,—I was very sorry you should take the trouble of cutting me such a nice piece of bread and butter, yesterday. I would of taken it but all of them saw you send it, and then they would have made enough to have talked about. But I should be very glad if you would cut me a nice piece of crust and put it in a piece of paper and send it, or else bring it, so that they do not see it, for they all watch me very much, and I should like to be your friend and you to be mine. Mrs. Winslow, (the nurse) is going to chapel. I will make it up with you when I can go as far. Do not send it if you cannot spare it. Good bye, and God bless you.' Although she prevaricated about this letter, she appears to have gradually improved from this time on, and one day walked out of the hospital and left it altogether. She subsequently wrote a letter to the authorities expressing her regret at having gone on as she did."

One of the most remarkable instances of the kind, is that of Sarah Jacob, known as the "Welsh Fasting Girl," and whose history and tragical death excited a great deal of comment in the medical and lay press in Great Britain a few years ago. The following account of the case is mainly derived from Dr. Fowler's[10] interesting work.

Sarah Jacob was born May 12th, 1857. Her parents were farmers and were uneducated, simple-minded, and ignorant persons. In her earlier years she had been healthy, was intelligent, given to religious reading, and was said to have written poetry of her own composition. She was a very pretty child and was, according to the testimony of the vicar, the Rev. Evan Jones, a "good girl."

About February 15th, 1867, when she was not quite ten years of age, she complained of pain in the pit of the stomach, and one morning on getting up, she told her mother that she had found her mouth full of bloody froth. The pain continued, and medical attendance was obtained. Soon afterwards she had strong convulsions of an epileptiform character and then other spasms of a clearly hysterical form, during which her body was bent in the form of a bow as in tetanus, the head and heels only touching the bed. Then the muscular spasm ceased and she fell at full length on the bed. For a whole month she continued in a state of unconsciousness, suffering from frequent repetitions of severe convulsive attacks, during which time she took little food. Mr. Davies, the surgeon, said in his evidence, that she was for a whole month, in a kind of permanent fit, lying on her back, with rigidity of all the muscles. For some time her life was despaired of, then her fits ceased to be convulsive and consisted of short periods of loss of consciousness with sudden awakings. For the next two or three months (till August, 1867) she took daily, from six, gradually decreasing to four, teacupfuls of rice and milk, or oatmeal and milk, which according to her father's account, was cast up again immediately and blood and froth with it. During this time the bowels were only acted on once in six or nine days. "Up to this time," said her father, "she could move both arms and one leg, but the other leg was rigid."

By the beginning of October, 1867, her quantity of daily food had, it was affirmed, dwindled down to nothing but a little apple about the size of a pill, which she took from a tea-spoon. At this time she made water about every other day; she looked very bad in the face, but was not thin. On the tenth day of October, it was solemnly declared that she ceased to take any food whatever, and so continued till the day of her death, December 17th, 1869, a period of two years, two months, and one week.

"Of the veracity of the assertion in respect of *the one week*," says Dr. Fowler, "there is unfortunately plenty of evidence. To the absurdity of believing in the barest possibility of twenty-six months absolute abstinence, it is sufficient to reply that when to our knowledge, she was completely deprived of food, the girl died! The parents most persistently impressed upon every private as well as official visitor, both before and during the last fatal watching, that the girl did not take food; that she could not swallow; that whenever food was mentioned to her she became as it were, excited;

that when it was offered to her she would have a fit, or the offer would make her ill. The sworn testimony of the vicar, the Rev. Wm. Thomas, Sister Clinch, Ann Jones, and the other nurses, is sufficiently confirmative on this point. Furthermore, the parents went so far as to expressly forbid the mere mention of food in the girl's presence."

Towards the end of October, 1867, the case had attracted so much attention that the inhabitants in the neighborhood first began visiting the marvellous little girl.

"In the beginning of November of the same year, the Rev. Evan Jones, B.D., the vicar of the parish, was sent for by the parents to visit Sarah Jacob. He was at once—by the mother—told of the girl's wonderful fasting powers; it was admitted she took water occasionally. He was also informed of the extraordinary perversion of her natural functions (the suppression of urine and fæcal evacuations.) He found her lying on her back in bed, which was covered with books. There was nothing then remarkable about her dress. The girl looked weak and delicate, though not pale, and answered only in monosyllables. 'The mother said her child was very anxious about the state of her soul, that it had such an effect upon her mind that she could not sleep.' I asked her myself if she had a desire to become a member of the Church of England? She said, 'Yes!' She continued to express that wish until July, 1869. At this time the reverend gentleman did not believe in the statements relative to the girl's abstinence. 'Every time,' he says, 'that I had a conversation with her up to the end of 1868, the parents both persisted that she lived without food, and continued their statements in January and February, 1869. I remonstrated with them and dwelt upon the apparent impossibility of the thing. They still persisted that it was a fact.'

"Even as late as September, 1869, the vicar reiterated his ministerial remonstrances. When, in the beginning of the spring of 1869, he observed the fantastical changes the parents made in the girl's daily attire, he told them about the remarks made in the papers about this dressing and dwelt upon the impropriety of it. They replied, 'She had no other pleasure—they did not like denying it to her.' During the following summer, finding that the girl looked more plump in the face and that her general improvement was more conspicuous, he said, 'Sarah is evidently improving and gaining, and you say she takes no food; you are certainly imposing on the public.' I then dwelt on the sinfulness of continuing the fraud on the public. I said there were on record several cases of alleged fasting, some of which had been put to the test and had been discovered to be impositions; that those families would ever be held in execration by posterity, and such would be the case with them whenever this imposture was found out. The mother then assured me no imposition would be discovered in that house, because there was none."

The father and mother both said that the Lord provided for her in a most natural way, and that it was a miracle. The father always talked about the "Doctor Mawr," meaning God Almighty; that she was supported by that "Big Doctor."

Then soon began the custom of leaving money or other presents with the child, till at last every one who visited her, was expected to give something. Open house was kept and pilgrims came from near and far to see the wonderful girl who lived without food.

When money was not forthcoming, presents of clothes, finery, books, or flowers, appear to have been substituted. Advantage was taken of these presents to bedeck the child in every variety of smartness. At one time she had a victorine about her neck and a wreath about her hair, then again, ornaments and a jacket on, and her hair neatly dressed with ribbons. At another time she had a silk shawl, a victorine around her neck, a small crucifix attached to a necklace, and little ribbons above the wrists. She had drab gloves on and her bed was nearly covered with books.

Notwithstanding the alleged fasting, Sarah Jacob continued to improve in health.

And now comes an astounding feature of this most remarkable case. The vicar became convinced that the instance was one of real abstinence. A little hysterical girl twelve years of age, by her perseverance in lying, had actually succeeded in inducing an educated gentleman to accept the truth of her statements! The following letter which was published on the 19th of February, 1869, speaks for itself:—

"A STRANGE CASE.

"To the Editor of the *Welshman*.

"Sir: Allow me to invite the attention of your readers to a most extraordinary case. Sarah Jacob, a little girl twelve years of age, and daughter of Mr. Evan Jacob, Lletherneuadd, in this parish, has not partaken of a single grain of any kind of food whatever, during the last sixteen months. She did occasionally swallow a few drops of water during the first few months of this period; but now she does not even do that. She still looks pretty well in the face and continues in the possession of all her mental faculties. She is in this and several other respects, a wonderful little girl.

"Medical men persist in saying that the thing is quite impossible, but all the nearest neighbors, who are thoroughly acquainted with the circumstances of the case, entertain no doubt whatever of the subject, and I am myself of the same opinion.

"Would it not be worth their while for medical men to make an investigation into the nature of this strange case? Mr. Evan Jacob would readily admit into his house any respectable person who might be anxious to watch it and to see for himself.

"I may add, that Lletherneuadd is a farm-house about a mile from New Inn, in this parish.

"Yours faithfully,
"THE VICAR OF LLANFIHANGEL-AR-ARTH."

The suggestions of the vicar relative to an investigation, were soon after afterwards acted upon by certain gentlemen of the neighborhood. A public meeting was called and a committee of watchers was appointed to be constantly in attendance in the room with Sarah Jacob, and to observe to the best of their ability, whether or not she took any food during the investigation. It was agreed that the watching was to continue for a fortnight.

Prior to the beginning of this watching, no precautions were taken against food being conveyed into the room and concealed there. The parents actually debarred the watchers from touching the child's bed. The very first element of success was therefore denied, and no wonder that the whole affair was subsequently regarded as an absurdity. The watching consisted in two different men taking alternate watches from eight till eight. The watching to see whether the child partook of food, commenced on March 22d, and ended April 5th, 1869—a period of fourteen days.

During the above fortnight, one of the watchers, in turn, was always close to her bed, and in her sight day and night, and at the time the bed was being made, which was generally every other morning, the four persons were always present and had every article thoroughly examined. The parents were allowed to go near the bed, as also was the little sister, six years old, who had been Sarah's constant companion and bed-fellow.

On Wednesday, April 7th, 1869, a public meeting was held at the Eagle Inn, Llandyfeil, to hear the statements of the parents and of the several persons who had watched the child during the fourteen days. The parents briefly detailed the condition and symptoms of their daughter from the commencement of her illness. At no time during the whole fourteen days did the pulse ever reach above ninety per minute, although exceedingly changeable, as it always had been. The following evidence was received from the watchers, and it is *said* that their statements were duly verified on oath before a magistrate:—

Watcher No. 1 said: I, Evan Edward Smith, watched Sarah Jacob for two consecutive nights, (*i. e.*, nights 22d and 23d of March) at the request of Mr. H. H. Davies, surgeon. The parents gave every facility to investigate the matter. I watched her with all possible care, and found nothing to suspect that food or drink was given her by foul means. I am quite sure she had nothing during my watch. I was dismissed on account of being suspected to doze on the second night.

Watcher No. 2. This watcher watched Sarah Jacob for a whole fortnight, and found no indications that the child had anything to eat or drink. He was a college student, Daniel Harris Davies.

Watcher No. 3. John Jones, a shopkeeper, gave similar evidence. He was a decided sceptic before he began watching, but after twelve days was thoroughly convinced of the fact that nothing in the shape of nourishment was given to the poor child. He watched every movement of all the inmates, and found nothing that would lead him to suspect that any nourishment was given to the little girl.

Watcher No. 4. James Harris Davies, a medical student, spoke in like manner, and was perfectly positive that nothing had been given to her during the fortnight he had watched there, with the exception of three drops of water, once, to moisten her lips with. He was as great a sceptic as any one before he began watching, but as he saw nothing to confirm his suspicions, he could conscientiously say that nothing had been given her during his watch.

Watcher No. 5. Evan Davies, of Powel Castle, who only watched her for one day, gave similar evidence, but as he was a neighbour he was dismissed for a stranger.

Watcher No. 6. Herbert Jones, watched only one day, and spoke in a similar manner, and was dismissed on account of his credulity.

Watcher No. 7. Thomas Davies, who had been the greatest sceptic of all, was strongly convinced. He watched Sarah Jacob twelve days, and was quite positive that nothing could have been given her during his watch. He watched her with all possible care, and was very cautious to be in a prominent place, where Sarah Jacob's mouth was always in sight.

Evidence, however, was given which went to show that the watching was very imperfectly performed; that occasionally the watchers left before their time had expired; that intoxicating liquors were taken by them to the house, and that one of them was drunk while there. It was also shown that the father and mother had free access to the bed, while the watchers were absolutely prohibited from examining it. It is therefore with entire justification that Dr. Fowler states that the watching "was the greatest possible farce and mockery."

After the report of the watchers the notoriety of Sarah Jacob of course became still greater; crowds came to visit her, and among others the Rev.

Frederic Rowland Young went to see her, and made an unsuccessful effort to cure her by laying on of hands. When Dr. Fowler visited her, August 30th, 1869, on getting out at the nearest railway station, he was met by little boys bearing placards with the words "Fasting Girl," and "This is the shortest way to Llethernoryadd-ucha," on them. In his letter to the *Times*, giving an account of his visit, Dr. Fowler says:—

"The first impression was most unfavorable, and to a medical man the appearances were most suspicious. The child was lying on a bed decorated as a bride, having around her head a wreath of flowers, from which was suspended a smart ribbon, the ends of which were joined by a small bunch of flowers, after the present fashion of ladies' bonnet strings. Before her, at proper reading distance, was an open Welsh book, supported by two other books on her body. The blanket covering was clean, tidy, and perfectly smooth. Across the fire-place, which was nearly opposite the foot of her bed, was an arrangement of shelves, well stocked with English and Welsh books, the gifts of various visitors to the house. The child is thirteen years of age, and is undoubtedly very pretty. Her face was plump, and her cheeks and lips of a beautiful rosy color. Her eyes were bright and sparkling, the pupils were very dilated, in a measure explicable by the fact of the child's head and face being shaded from the window-light by the projecting side of the cupboard bedstead. There was that restless movement and frequent looking out at the corners of the eyes so characteristic of simulative disease. Considering the lengthened inactivity of the girl, her muscular development was very good, and the amount of fat layer not inconsiderable. My friend stated that she looked even better than she did about a twelvemonth ago. There was a slight perspiration over the surface of the body. The pulse was perfectly natural, as were also the sounds of the lungs and heart, so far as I was enabled to make a stethoscopic examination. Having received permission to do this, I proceeded to make the necessary derangement of dress, when the girl went off into what the mother called a fainting fit. This consisted of nothing but a little and momentary hysterical crying and sobbing. The color never left the lips or cheeks. The pulse remained of the same power. Consciousness could have been but slightly diminished, inasmuch as on my then opening the eyelids I perceived a distinct upward and other movement of the eyeballs. Each percussion stroke of my examination, and even the pressure of the stethoscope, produced an expression of pain, which elicited a natural sympathy from the mother, and an assertion that a continuance of such examination would bring on further fits. On percussing the region of the stomach, I most distinctly perceived the sound of gurgling, which we know to be caused by the admixture of air and fluid in motion. The most positive assertion of the parents was subsequently made that saving a fortnightly moistening of her lips with cold water, the child had neither ate nor drank anything for the last twenty-three months. The whole region of the belly was tympanitic, and the muscular walls of this cavity were tense and drum-like—a condition not infrequently concomitant of a well-known class of nervous disorders. The child's intellectual faculties and special senses were perfectly healthy. Before her illness she was very much devoted to religious reading. This devotion has lately considerably increased. She is a member of the Church of England, and has been confirmed."

Dr. Fowler then adds some other interesting particulars, all going to show the impossibility of the girl's being the subject of any exhausting disease, or of even having been continuously in bed, as her parents asserted, for nearly two years; and then says:—

"The whole case is in fact one of simulative hysteria, in a young girl having the propensity to deceive very strongly developed. Therewith may be probably associated the power or habit of prolonged fasting. Both patient and mother admitted the occasional occurrence of the choking sensation called *globus hystericus*."

This letter excited renewed discussion in the newspapers, and a second public meeting was called to make arrangements for a second watching. At this meeting it was decided to bring down from Guy's Hospital, London, several trained nurses, who were to conduct the watching; and the following resolutions were adopted, as expressing the terms under which the inquiry was to be conducted:—

1. It would be advisable, before taking any steps in the matter, to obtain a written legal guarantee from the father of Sarah Jacob sanctioning the necessary proceedings. 2. That the duty of the nurses shall be to watch Sarah Jacob with a view to ascertain whether she partakes of any kind of food, and at the end of a fortnight to report upon the case before the local

committee in Carmarthenshire, and, if required, at Guy's Hospital. 3. That two nurses shall be constantly awake and on the watch in the girl's room, night and day. 4. It would be advisable for the nearest medical practitioner to watch the progress of the case; and it will be absolutely necessary for him to *be prepared against any serious symptoms of exhaustion, supervening on the strict enforcement of the watching, and to act according to his judgment.* 5. That the room in which the girl sleeps shall be bared of all unnecessary furniture, and all possible places in the room for the concealment of food shall be closed and kept under the continual scrutiny of the watchers. 6. That if considered desirable by the local medical practitioner, or by the nurses, the bedstead on which the girl now lies shall be replaced by a single iron one. 7. That the bed on which the parents now sleep, in Sarah Jacob's room, shall be given up absolutely to the nurses. 8. That the parents be not allowed to sleep in the same room as the girl; that if they cannot at all times be prevented from approaching her, they should be previously searched (their pockets and other recesses of clothing as well as the interior of their mouths); and that no wetted towels or other such articles be allowed to be used about the girl by the parents, or any other person save the nurses; that the children of the family, and in fact every other person whatever (except the nurses), have similar restraints put upon them. 9. That the nurses have the sole management of preparing the room, bed, and patient, prior to the commencement of the watching. 10. That, as it is asserted the action of the bowels and bladder is entirely suspended, special attention must be directed to these organs.

Four experienced women nurses were accordingly deputed from Guy's Hospital to take the entire charge of Sarah Jacob, and to watch her for fourteen days. They were instructed not to prevent her having food if she asked for it, but they were to see that she got none without their knowledge. On the 9th of December, 1869, at 4 P.M., the room was cleared of people and the watching began.

In the first place it was ascertained that the girl had repeated evacuations of urine, and once, at least, of fæces.

Gradually evidences of mental and physical disturbance began to appear. The watch was so closely kept that no food or drink reached the child, and she did not ask for any.

"At 10 P.M.," to quote the language of the journal kept by the sister nurse, "she was restless and threw her arms about. She was very cold, and the nurses put warm flannels on her. This was the last day on which she passed urine."

Thursday, December 16, 3 A.M.—She was rolling from one side of the bed to the other. At half-past three she wished the bed made, and they made it. She was looking very pale and anxious. Her eyes were sunk and her nose pinched, and the cheek bones were prominent. Her arms and hands were cold, her feet and legs were the same. Ann Jones, one of the nurses, says in her memoranda, "She was very restless and appeared to me to be sinking. Her lips were very dry, and her mouth seemed parched." The peculiar smell (the starvation smell) about the bed was so strong as to make the sister nurse quite ill.

At 11 A.M., the vicar saw her and told the parents that the child was gradually failing, and suggested to them the propriety of sending the nurses away and giving her a chance to obtain food, but they refused, saying that there was nothing to do but what the nurses were doing, and that they had seen her quite as weak before. The parents were urged by others to give up the fight by sending the nurses away, but they refused on the ground that want of food had nothing to do with the symptoms, and that she would not eat whether the nurses were there or not.

Ann Jones subsequently testified before the coroner: "Before one and two o'clock on Thursday afternoon (Dec. 16), she kept talking to herself. I could not understand whether she was speaking Welsh or English. Up to that time I could understand her. She pointed her fingers at some books; I gave her one, but she took no notice of it; she was not able to read it. *Both parents were then told the girl was dying.*"

Repeatedly they were begged to withdraw the nurses, and again and again they refused, saying there was no occasion—that she had often been in that way, that it was not from want of food, etc. The girl became weaker and weaker; low, muttering delirium ensued, and on the 17th of December, 1869, at about half-past three o'clock, P.M., the "Welsh Fasting Girl" died, actually starved to death, in the middle of the nineteenth century and in one of the most Christian and civilized countries of the world!

But this was not the end. Public opinion was much excited both against those who had sanctioned and conducted what appeared to have been a senseless and cruel experiment, and against the father and mother who had wilfully and persistently refused to allow food to be given to the dying child. A coroner's inquest was held, and the coroner appears to have made a very satisfactory charge to the jury after the rendition of the testimony. He said there could be no doubt of the child having died of starvation, and that the responsibility rested with the father, who had knowingly and designedly failed to cause his child to take food. The mother was not responsible unless it could be shown that she had been given food for the child by the father, and had withheld it from her. It was marvellous, he said, how the father could have made out such a story—such a hideous mass of nonsense, as he had under oath attempted to impose on the jury.

The jury deliberated for a quarter of an hour, and then returned a verdict of "Died from starvation, caused by negligence to induce the child to take food on the part of the father;" which constituted manslaughter.

Evan Jacob was therefore arrested. But the Secretary of State for the Home Department took the matter up and determined that the proceedings should go farther than the local authorities intended. At first it was contemplated to indict the members of the General Committee for conspiracy, but it was finally concluded to include only the medical gentlemen who had accepted the responsibility of superintending the watching, as well as both parents of the deceased child.

The initial proceeding took place before a full bench of magistrates, and continued eight days. The Crown and the accused had eminent counsel, and many witnesses were examined. At the conclusion of the inquiry the presiding magistrate announced that it had been determined by the court that no case had been made out against the physicians, who had not been shown to have undertaken any other duty than that of advising the nurses, and that it did not appear that their advice had been asked. As to the father and mother the court had decided to send them both for trial for manslaughter, at the next assizes. In due time they were arraigned, they pleaded not guilty, but after being defended by able counsel, the jury, after an absence of about half an hour, returned with a verdict of guilty against both the prisoners, but with a recommendation of the mother to the merciful consideration of the court, on the ground that she was under the control of her husband. The man protested his innocence, and the woman "buried her face in her shawl and wept bitterly."

His Lordship, in passing sentence, said: "Prisoners at the bar, you have been found guilty of a most aggravated offence. I entirely concur with the verdict which the jury have given, and I shall act upon the recommendation which they have presented in favor of the female prisoner, the mother, though, I must say, that I cannot but feel that it is a greater crime in the mother than the father, since it is more contrary to the common nature of mothers, to neglect their children in the manner in which you have treated this unfortunate child. It is contrary to the nature, even, of a father. But I shall act upon the recommendation of the jury, upon the ground they have put forward, that you have been subject to the control of your husband more than has appeared from the evidence of the case. But the offence is, as I have said, a serious one, on this ground; that there can be no doubt that both of you have persisted in this fraudulent deception, upon your neighbors, and upon the public, and that in order to carry out that fraudulent deception and to preserve yourselves from detection you were willing to risk the life of that child. The life of that child has been lost in that wicked experiment which you tried. Therefore, the sentence that I shall inflict on you, Evan Jacob, is, that you be imprisoned and kept at hard labor for twelve calendar months; and that upon you, Hannah Jacob, will be more lenient in consideration of the recommendation of the jury, and it is, that you be imprisoned and kept to hard labor for the period of six calendar months."

Thus ended one of the most remarkable and interesting histories of human folly, credulity, and criminality which the present day has produced. Comment upon its teaching is scarcely necessary; but the thoughtful reader will not fail to perceive how important a bearing it has upon the whole subject of belief without full and free inquiry, and that how all the facts which science has gathered during ages of painful labor, go for naught, even with educated persons, when brought face to face with the false assertions of a hysterical girl, and of two ignorant and deceitful peasants. If there is any one thing we know, it is that there can be no force without the metamorphosis of matter of some kind. Here was a girl maintaining her weight—actually growing—her animal heat kept at its due standard, her mind active, her heart beating, her lungs respiring, her skin exhaling, her limbs moving whenever she wished them to move, and all, as very many persons supposed, without the ingestion of the material by which alone such things could be. And yet such is the tendency of the average human mind to be deceived, that it would be perfectly possible to re-enact in the city of New York the whole tragedy of Sarah Jacob, should ever a hysterical girl take it into head to do so; and there would not be wanting, even from among those who might read this history, individuals who would credit any monstrous declarations she might make. Even now in a little town in Belgium, an ecstatic girl is going through the same performance with extraordinary additions, and books are written by learned physicians and theologians, with the object of establishing the truth of her pretensions. To this most remarkable instance, and one other of similar though perhaps even more remarkable characteristic, the attention of the reader will presently be invited. But in view of these things one is almost tempted to say with Cardinal Carafa, "*Quandoquidem populus decipi vult, decipiatur.*"

FOOTNOTES:

[3] "De puella quæ sine cibo et potu vitam transigit." Parisiis Ann. MDXLII.

[4] "Παρατηρήσεων sive observationum medicarum, rararum, novarum, admirabilium, et monstrosarum. Volumen, tomis septem de toto homine institutum." Lugduni 1606, p. 306.

These cases are cited by Wanley in his "Wonders of the Little World," but I have taken care in most instances to refer to the originals, several of which are in my library.

[5] "Wonders of the Little World." London, 1806, p. 375.

[6] Opuscula Medica. Parisiis, 1639, pp. 64, 65, 66.

[7] Observationum et curationum chirurgicarum, centuria secunda. Genevæ, 1611, p. 116.

[8] Wonderful Characters: By Henry Wilson and James Caulfield. London.

[9] British Medical Journal, July 16, 1870.

[10] A complete History of the Welsh Fasting Girl (Sarah Jacob,) with Comments thereon, and Observations on Death from Starvation. London, 1871.

III.

ABSTINENCE FROM FOOD WITH STIGMATIZATION.

One hundred and fifty-three persons have at one time or another, according to Dr. Imbert-Gourbeyre,[11] received the stigmata; that is, been marked in a miraculous manner with the wounds received by Christ at the crucifixion. Of these, eight, are according to the same authority now living, and two assert that they do not eat. I propose to consider at some length the main points in the histories of these two, Palma d'Oria and Louise Lateau, and in so doing I shall avail myself of the works of those, who are firm believers in the miraculous interposition of God to produce the effects, of which they are said to be the subjects. These cases are very little known in this country. Instances of the kind are extremely rare among practical common sense nations, like those inhabiting the British Isles, and their descendants in America. Of the whole one hundred and fifty-three cases recorded by Dr. Imbert-Gourbeyre, but one—Jane Gray—was British, and hers is the most doubtful case in the list, for the fact rests only on the testimony of one Thomas Bourchier, an English minor brother, who asserts that she had the stigmata in the feet. Of the remainder, the very large majority are of Italy, and as Dr. Imbert-Gourbeyre says:

"Quel pays fut jamais si fertile en miracles?"[12]

To the account of a visit made to Oria for the purpose of studying the phenomena exhibited by Palma, made by Dr. Imbert-Gourbeyre, I am indebted for the following details:

Palma, at the time of the visit in 1871, was sixty-six years old, humpbacked, thin, small, and with light, expressive eyes. For several years she had not left the house, and was, on account of her sufferings, scarcely able to walk. Occasionally, when she felt particularly well, she took a few steps about the room supported by a cane. In her youth she had been very strong and active.

At the first interview, after some conversation in the course of which Palma declared that she had often seen Louise Lateau while in ecstasy, the doctor directed the conversation towards the subject of hallucination. While thus engaged and seated close to Palma, he felt her strike him gently on the arm, and at the same time saw the abbé, who had come with him, fall on his knees. He turned toward Palma; her eyes were closed, her hands clasped, her mouth wide open, and on her tongue he saw the host—the body of Christ. Immediately, he fell on his knees also, and worshipped it. Palma protruded her tongue still farther, as if she wanted to give him every opportunity of seeing that the host was really there; then she ate it, closed her mouth and remained perfectly quiet on the sofa upon which she was reclining. It was then almost four o'clock in the afternoon, the day was fading, the room was badly lit by a little window, high from the floor. The miraculous host appeared to him to be as white as wax, and somewhat thick. On account of the little light, and the short time that this extraordinary communion lasted, he was unable to determine whether or not it was marked according to the custom of the church.

In regard to this wonderful event—that is, if it be not a fact viewed unequally—it is further to be said that Palma disclosed to Dr. Imbert-Gourbeyre, that two or three times, the holy element, which be it remembered is believed by the great majority of Christians to be the real body of Christ, was brought to her by the devil, and that then she refused it. Sometimes he had the figure of an angel, but she knew him by the sign of reprobation which he wore on his forehead—a little horn. Moreover she saw that the wicked creature hesitated, and was a little embarrassed. She intoned the *Gloria Patri*, and made the sign of the cross, and he instantly took flight and disappeared. In order to ascertain what it all meant, her confessor forbade her to receive the miraculous communion for eight days. Hardly had that period expired when Jesus Christ himself brought her the communion. Before giving it to her he made her recite the *Gloria Patri* three times. Then he said to her, "Have I fled as the demon did? No. Therefore reassure yourself. It is really I."

These miraculous circumstances had been going on for about two years when Dr. Imbert-Gourbeyre made his visit to Palma. Sometimes it was brought to her by Christ, as in the instance specified, or by some saint, as St. Peter, St. Vincent de Paul, St. Francis d'Assisi, in the company of her guardian angel, and other saints and angels. At other times it was brought by priests and confessors of the olden time, long since dead.

An Italian bishop stated, that at the moment of the miraculous sacrament on one occasion, he had seen the host flying through the air before entering Palma's mouth, but the doctor questioned her attendant on this point, and she declared that she had not seen that, and she assured him that the host was never seen by any one till it rested on Palma's tongue. The doctor inclines to the belief that the attendant was right, but he states that nevertheless a French apostolic missionary had asserted that he had seen the same thing.

Well, if the consecrated bread be really the body of Christ that was given for the salvation of the world, what horrible blasphemy to state such things of it, what vileness to believe them, what a barefaced imputation on the reason of man to spread these shocking details before him and ask him to accept them as true of the God he worships!

After witnessing the communion, Dr. Imbert-Gourbeyre was requested to withdraw into the adjoining room, while Palma got ready for her other performances. In a few minutes he was informed that all was in order. One of the women went in first and returning immediately, the others were invited to enter. The stigmatization had already begun on the forehead. He saw a stream of blood flowing from the left frontal eminence along the side of the nose. A handkerchief was given to Palma; she held it to her nose for a moment and the hæmorrhage soon stopped. He examined the blood and found that it did not differ in appearance, color or temperature from ordinary blood. He then examined the handkerchief, and besides numerous rotund spots he perceived other figures resembling hearts, with stains of blood proceeding from them, indicating the flames of love. All this appeared to him to be very extraordinary, for though he had often seen people bleed from the nose, he had never seen them bleed like that.

After this incident Palma continued the performances—*actions de grace* he calls them—her hands clasped and her eyes closed. In the lower limbs, especially the left, there was a tremor like a nervous trembling which was soon quieted. After a few minutes she rubbed her hands together, made the sign of the cross and returned naturally to the conversation. He then examined her forehead and endeavored to ascertain where the blood had come from. The skin was intact without the least opening. She showed him above the right frontal eminence a hole in the cranium, from which at a former period, five little pieces of bone had been discharged. The opening was entirely covered over by the scalp, and he was surprised to find that there was no cicatrix. It was round, the end of his index finger entered it readily, and it was just such an opening as would have been produced by the crown of a trephine. At the time it was made, the skin opened to allow of the exit of the pieces of bone; then it closed without leaving the trace of a scar. It was the same with the stigmata. They closed at once without there being any marks to indicate the place whence the blood had flowed. This hole in the skull had been caused by some particular circumstances that no one was willing to reveal to him, but which he says are reported in the journal of the directors of this woman, and which will soon be published. Most medical men will come to the conclusion that it was due to caries and necrosis of the bone, of syphilitic origin.

During another visit Palma told Dr. Imbert-Gourbeyre that she had eaten nothing for seven years, but that she was obliged to drink frequently on account of the great internal heat, which like a fire consumed her. She then drank in his presence two carafes of water at one time, and the doctor states that "this water became so hot in her stomach that it was vomited boiling. She also had often ejected from her mouth oil, and another fluid of a balsamic character, in which, on standing for some time, bodies resembling the consecrated host were formed."

The doctor then relates the following details, which I give in his own words, in further illustration of the character of his mental organization and of the pretensions put forth by the woman, whose word seems to have been sufficient to convince him of anything at all, no matter how preposterous. Four years previously he had been so unfortunate as to lose by death his eldest child:

"A year after his death, I had met a woman of great renown for piety, and who was even regarded as a receiver of celestial communications. I had commended my poor Joseph to her. Some time after she assured me that my son was saved, and that he was in paradise. She declared that in a vision she had seen him near our Lord; he was happy. Various circumstances, which it is useless to mention here, had caused me to believe in the truth of this asserted revelation. Being in Oria, I wished to have as much certainty as possible in regard to the matter, and as I knew that Palma was in spiritual communication with many pious souls scattered over the earth, I said to her in the course of our conversation, 'tell me, Palma, do you know M. —— de X——,' giving her the baptismal name of the woman in question. 'No sir,' she answered. I then related to her my history in detail, taking care not to ask her opinion in advance, although I felt sure that she would explain the thing to me. She listened with the utmost attention to the superioress who translated my words, and when Mother Becaud came to say that the woman had had a vision of my son, and that he was in paradise, Palma stretched out her arm in a solemn manner as a sign of negative, and said to me, 'He is saved, but he is still in purgatory.'

"'Is it possible? Palma,' I cried, profoundly moved: 'Since you tell me this, you are in conscience bound to get him out of that place of expiation as soon as possible, and I commend him immediately to your prayers.'

"'Yes, sir,' she said, 'I will pray for him, and when I am sure of his deliverance, I will send you word by Father de Pace.'

"The following morning at my visit I again commended my poor child to Palma, and on the following Friday evening on taking leave of her, I asked if she had prayed that morning for my son, 'No sir,' she answered. 'I will only do so on the day of All Saints.' 'Then,' said I to Palma, 'will you allow madame the superioress to take the answer?' 'Very willingly,' said the seeress. On the 7th of November, I received at Nice the following letter:

> "'SIR,
>
> "'I have fulfilled the promise which I made to you in accordance with your wish to go to Palma on All Saints Day, in order to ascertain whether or not your wishes in regard to your son had been granted. That good soul assured me twice that he had gone to heaven that very morning, God be praised a thousand times!
>
> "'Thus sir, I have done what I could for your consolation.

>"'I have the honor to be, etc.
>
>"'Sister Marie Becaud.'

"This letter was post marked at Oria, November 2d."

I should not venture to insult the intelligence of the reader with these idiotic details but for the reasons stated, and additionally, that they carry conviction with them to thousands of minds, honest doubtless, but which are accustomed to grovel in superstition, and falsehood, which they are unable to test by right standards.

A phase in Palma's spiritual pathology has been alluded to cursorily, but has not yet been considered with the fulness proper in connection with stigmatization, and that is the occurrence of hæmorrhagic spots on various parts of her body, and which she so managed as to convey the idea that they were symbolical of various holy things. On the back of her hand she convinced Dr. Imbert-Gourbeyre that she bled in the shape of the cross, and he gives a wood-cut representing a cross on the dorsum of the hand, a little above the space between the first and second fingers. This is surrounded by other rectilinear figures. On her breast and back, other figures were obtained by placing handkerchiefs on the parts. The doctor thus procured several mementoes of his visit, in the shape of pieces of linen stained with spots of blood somewhat resembling hearts, with flames coming out of them, suns, roses, crosses, etc. He gives several plates in his book representing these figures, of the reality of the miraculous formation of which he has not the slightest doubt.

Another phenomenon has also been mentioned incidentally, and that is the intense heat which Palma declared she felt, and which the doctor refers to as the "divine fire." He had brought with him from Paris, a thermometer to use in determining the extraordinary temperature of this fire. He examined her with this instrument while she felt this divine fire, but failed to find any abnormal increase; her pulse at the time was 72. "I made this experiment," he says, "to satisfy my scientific conscience, [God save the mark!] but I ought to say that I was ashamed of myself for presuming to measure this divine fire by such an instrument." He is right, science is not for him, or those like him.

On one occasion while Palma was in ecstasy, Antonietta, who was near her, laid bare her chest a little, and cried with enthusiasm, "she is burning!" Dr. Imbert-Gourbeyre approached and smelt something like the burning of linen. The dress was opened and her chemise was found to be burnt on the left side just over the collar bone, and immediately below this, scorched in the shape of "a magnificent emblem representing a monstrance. The fire was invisible, but its traces were very evident."

In a note he states that it was affirmed that Palma's temperature on similar occasions had reached 100° centigrade, (212° Fahrenheit) a fact which he does not doubt, although his thermometer did not show it. "That her chemise," he says, "burnt by invisible fire, which escaped the thermometer, was more extraordinary than if the instrument had indicated a temperature of 100°."

I shall not stop now to comment further on the circumstances detailed by Dr. Imbert-Gourbeyre, and of which I have cited but a small part. I will only say at present that science and common sense would conclude in regard to Palma d'Oria,

1st. That she had probably at a former period contracted syphilis.

2d. That she was strongly hysterical.

3d. That she was the subject of purpura hæmorrhagica.

4th. That she was a most unmitigated humbug and liar.

And now we come to the consideration of a case of stigmatization which has greatly stirred both the theological and the scientific world of Europe—that of Louise Lateau—and here again I shall draw largely, though by no means exclusively, from the works of the believers in the miraculous production of the phenomena manifested.[13]

Louise Lateau was born at Bois-d'Haine, a small village in Belgium, on the 30th of January, 1850. She was reared in the utmost poverty, was chlorotic, and did not menstruate till she was eighteen years old. She loved solitude and silence, and when not engaged in work—and she does not appear to have labored much—she spent her time in meditation and prayer. She was subject to paroxysms of ecstasy, during which, as many other ecstasies, she spoke very edifying things, of charity, poverty, and the priesthood. She saw St. Ursula, St. Roch, St. Theresa, and the Holy Virgin. Persons who saw her in these states declared that, while lying on the bed, her whole body was raised up more than a foot high, the heels alone being in contact with the bed.

The stigmatization ensued very soon after these seizures. On a Friday she bled from the left side of her chest. On the following Friday this flow was renewed, and in addition, blood escaped from the dorsal surfaces of both feet; and on the third Friday, not only did she bleed from the side and feet, but also from the dorsal and palmar surface of both hands. Every succeeding Friday the blood flowed from these places, and finally other points of exit were established on the forehead and between the shoulders.

At first these bleedings only took place at night, but after two or three months they occurred in the daytime, and were accompanied by paroxysms of ecstasy, during which she was insensible to all external impressions, and acted the passion of Jesus and the crucifixion.

M. Warlomont, being commissioned by the Royal Academy of Medicine of Belgium to examine Louise Lateau, went to her house, accompanied by several friends, and made a careful examination of her person. At that time, Friday morning at six o'clock, the blood was flowing freely from all the stigmata. In a few moments the sacrament would be brought to her, and then the second act of the drama would begin. The scene that followed can be best described in M. Warlomont's own words:

"It is a quarter-past six. 'Here comes the communion,' said M. Niels [a priest], 'kneel down.' Louise fell on her knees on the floor, closed her eyes and crossed her hands, on which the communion-cloth was extended. A priest, followed by several acolytes, entered; the penitent put out her tongue, received the holy wafer, and then remained immovable in the attitude of prayer.

"We observed her with more care than seemed to have been hitherto given to her at similar periods. Some thought that she was simply in a state of meditation, from which she would emerge in the course of half an hour or so. But it was a mistake. Having taken the communion, the penitent went into a special state. Her immobility was that of a statue, her eyes were closed; on raising the eyelids the pupils were seen to be largely dilated, immovable, and apparently insensible to light. Strong pressure made upon the parts in the vicinity of the stigmata caused no sensation of pain, although a few moments before they were exquisitely tender. Pricking the skin gave no evidence of the slightest sensibility. A limb, on being raised, offered no resistance, and sank slowly back to its former position. Anæsthesia was complete, unless the cornea remained still impressionable. The pulse had fallen from 120 to 100 pulsations. At a given moment I raised one of the eyelids, and M. Verriest quickly touched the cornea. Louise at once seemed to recover herself from a sound sleep, arose and walked to a chair, upon which she seated herself. 'This time,' I said, 'we have wakened her.' 'No,' said M. Niels, looking at his watch, 'it was time for her to awake.'"

She remained conscious; the blood still continued to flow; the anæsthesia had ceased, her pulse rose to 120, and at the end of half an hour she was herself. "Our first visit ended here. At half-past eleven we made another. The poor child had resumed her attitude of extreme suffering, against which she contended with all the energy that remained to her. The wounds in the hands still continued to bleed. M. Verriest auscultated with care the lungs, heart, and great vessels, and found the *bruit de souffle*, which he had detected in the morning at the apex of the heart and over the carotids. The handle of a spoon pressed against the velum, the base of the tongue, and the pharynx, provoked no effort at vomiting. The glasses of our spectacles, as they came in contact with the air expired, were covered with vapor. As the patient appeared to suffer from our presence, we went away.

"We made our third visit at two o'clock. There were still fifteen minutes before the beginning of the ecstatic crisis, which always took place punctually at a quarter past two and ended at about half past four. The pupils at this time were slightly contracted, the eyelids were almost entirely closed; the eyes, looking at nothing, were veiled from our view. We tried in vain to attract her attention; her mind was otherwise engaged, and her pains were evidently becoming more intense. At exactly a quarter past two her eyes became fixed in a direction above and to the right. The ecstasy had begun.

"The time had now come to introduce those who were prompted by curiosity. This could now be done without inconvenience, for the ecstatic, for the ensuing two hours, would be lost to the appreciation of what might be passing around her. The room crowded, could hold about ten persons, but enough were allowed to enter to make the total twenty-five. These placed themselves in two ranks, of which the front one kneeling, allowed the rear ones to see all that was going on. All this was done under the direction of M. le Curé, who took every pains to give us a good view of what was going to happen.

"Louise was seated on the edge of her chair; her body, inclined forward, seemed to wish to follow the direction of her eyes, which did not look, but were fixed on vacancy. Her eyes were opened to their fullest extent, of a dull, lustreless appearance, turned above and to the right, and of an absolute immobility. A few workings of the lids were now observed and became more frequent if the eyelids were touched. The pupils, largely dilated, showed very little sensibility to light, and all that remained of vision was shown by slight winking when the hand was suddenly brought close to the eyes. The whole face lacked expression. At certain moments, either spontaneously or as a consequence of divers provocations, a light smile, to which the muscles of the face generally did not contribute, wandered over her lips. Then the face resumed its primitive expression, and thus she remained for the half-hour which constituted the 'first station.'

"The 'second station' was that of genuflection. It had failed at one time, but had again appeared. The young girl fell on her knees, clasped her hands, and remained for about a quarter of an hour in the attitude of contemplation. Then she arose and again resumed her sitting posture.

"The 'third station' began at three o'clock. Louise inclined herself a little forward, raised her body slowly, and then extended herself at full length, face downward, on the floor. There was neither rigidity nor extreme precipitation; nothing in fact, calculated to produce injuries. The knees first supported her body, then it rested on these and the elbows, and finally her face was brought in actual close contact with the tiled floor. At first the head rested on the left arm, but very soon the patient made a quick and sudden movement, and the arms were extended from the body in the form of a cross. At the same time the feet were brought together so that the dorsum of the right was in contact with the sole of the left foot. This position did not vary for an hour and a half. When the end of the crisis approached, the arms were brought close to the sides of the body, then suddenly the poor girl rose to her knees, her face turns to the wall, her cheeks become colored, her eyes have regained their expression, her countenance expands, and the ecstasy is at an end."

Further particulars are given, and an apparatus was constructed and applied to Louise's hand and arm so as to prevent any external excitation of the hæmorrhage. It was apparently shown that there was no such interference, for the blood began to flow at the usual time on Friday.

In addition to the stigmata and the paroxysms of ecstasy, Louise declared that she did not sleep, had eaten or drank nothing for four years, had had no fæcal evacuation for three years and a half, and that the urine was entirely suppressed.

M. Warlomont examined the blood and products of respiration chemically, and satisfied himself of their normal character, except that the former contained an excessive amount of white corpuscles.

When being closely interrogated, Louise admitted that, though she did not sleep, she had short periods of forgetfulness at night. On M. Warlomont suddenly opening a cupboard in her room, he found it to contain fruit and bread, and her chamber communicated directly with a yard at the back of the house. It was therefore perfectly possible for her to have slept, eaten, defecated, and urinated, without any one knowing that she did so.

The conclusions arrived at by M. Warlomont were, that the stigmatizations and ecstasies of Louise Lateau were real and to be explained upon well-known physiological and pathological principles, that she "worked, and dispensed heat, that she lost every Friday a certain quantity of blood by the stigmata, that the air she expired contained the vapor of water and carbonic acid, that her weight had not materially altered since she had come under observation. She consumes carbon and it is not from her own body that she gets it. Where does she get it from? Physiology answers, 'She eats.'"

Relative to the assumed abstinence in the cases of Palma d'Oria, Louise Lateau and other subjects of ecstasy and stigmata, it is not necessary, in view of the remarks already made on this subject in a previous chapter, to devote further consideration to it here. The conclusion arrived at by M. Warlomont is the only one which science can tolerate. Should Louise Lateau or Palma d'Oria ever be subjected to as close watching as was the poor little Welsh Fasting Girl, Sarah Jacob, it will certainly terminate as badly for them as for her, unless they yield to the demands of nature and take the food which the organism requires.

FOOTNOTES:

[11] Les Stigmatisées; Palma d'Oria, etc. 2d Edition, Paris, 1873, p. 263.

[12] Op. cit., t. ii.

[13] For the theological view of this remarkable case the reader is referred to the following works, a part only of those written in support of her pretensions. "Louise Lateau de Bois-d'Haine, sa vie, ses extases, ses stigmates: étude Médicale," par le Dr. Lefebvre, Louvain, 1873. "Les stigmatisées; Louise Lateau, etc.," par le Docteur A. Imbert-Gourbeyre, Paris, 1873. "Biographie de Louise Lateau," par H. Van Looy, Tournai, Paris and Leipzig, 1874. "Louise Lateau de Bois-d'Haine etc.," par le Dr. A. Rohling, Paris, 1874. "Louise Lateau, ihr Wunderleben u.s.w.," Von Paul Majunke, Berlin, 1875.

Among the treatises in which the miracle is denied, and the phenomena attributed to either disease or fraud are; "Louise Lateau; Rapport Médical sur la stigmatisée de Bois-d'Haine, fait à l'académie royale de médecine de Belgique," par le Dr. Warlomont, Bruxelles and Paris, 1875. "Science et miracle, Louise Lateau, ou la stigmatisée Belge," par le Dr. Bourneville, Paris, 1875. "Les Miracles," par M. Virchow, Revue des cours scientifiques, January 23rd 1875.

IV.

THE BROOKLYN CASE.

For several years past there have been rumors more or less definite in character that a young lady in Brooklyn was not only living without food, but was possessed of some mysterious faculty by which she could foretell events, read communications without the aid of the eyes, and accurately describe occurrences in distant places, through clairvoyance or whatever other name may be applied to the influence.

Finally, in the *New York Herald* of October 20th, 1878, appeared an account, headed "Life without Food. An Invalid Lady who for fourteen years has lived without nourishment." As this account is apparently authentic, and as the statements made have never been contradicted, I do not hesitate to quote from it. Some of the letters which have appeared in response to a proposition I offered, and to which fuller reference will presently be made, have accused me of dragging the young lady before the public. It will be seen, however, that her friends and physicians are responsible for all the publicity given to the case.

Leaving out of consideration for the present the alleged marvellous endowments of this young lady, as regards seeing without her eyes, second sight, etc., I quote from the *Herald* the essential points relative to her clinical history and abstinence from food:

"In a modest, secluded house at the corner of Myrtle Avenue and Downing Street, Brooklyn, lives an invalid lady afflicted with paralysis, with a history so remarkable and extraordinary that, notwithstanding it is vouched for by physicians of standing, it is almost incredible. It is claimed that for a period of nearly fourteen years she has lived absolutely without food or nourishment of any kind. The case has been kept by the family of the patient a well guarded secret, it having led them to a strict seclusion as the only means of protection against the visits of the curious and incredulous.

"The name of the remarkable person is Miss Mollie Fancher. To the half dozen medical gentlemen who have seen and attended her, her case is inexplicable. To learn the history of the strange case a *Herald* reporter yesterday called on several persons familiar with the facts. The first person seen was Dr. Ormiston, of No. 74 Hanson Place, Brooklyn, who attended her. He said:—'It seems incredible, but from everything I can learn Mollie Fancher never eats. The elder Miss Fancher, her aunt, who takes care of her, is a lady of the highest intelligence. She was at one time quite wealthy, and she has at present a comfortable income. I have every reason to believe that her statements are in every detail reliable. During a dozen visits to the sick chamber I have never detected evidence of the patient having eaten a morsel.'"

After interviewing a lady intimate with the family, the reporter sought out Dr. Speir, the attending physician of the patient, and thus details his experience with that gentleman:

"Dr. Speir was found in his comfortable little office, and the errand of the writer made known:—

"'Is it true, Doctor, that a patient of yours has lived for fourteen years without taking food?'

"'If you refer to Miss Fancher, yes. She became my patient in 1864. Her case is a most remarkable one.'

"'But has she eaten nothing during all these years?'

"'I can safely say she has not.'

"'Are the family also willing to vouch for the truth of this extraordinary statement?'

"'You will find them very reticent to newspaper men and to strangers generally. I do not believe any food—that is, solids—ever passed the woman's lips since her attack of paralysis, consequent upon her mishap. As for an occasional teaspoonful of water or milk, I sometimes force her to take it by using an instrument to pry open her mouth, but that is painful to her. As early as 1865 I endeavored to sustain life in this way, for I feared that, in obedience to the universal law of nature, she would die of gradual inanition or exhaustion, which I thought would sooner or later ensue; but I was mistaken. The case knocks the bottom out of all existing medical theories, and is, in a word, miraculous.'

"'Did you ever,' asked the reporter, 'make an experiment to satisfy your professional accuracy in regard to her abstinence?'

"'Several times I have given her emetics on purpose to discover the truth; but the result always confirmed the statement that she had taken no food. It sounds strangely, but it is so. I have taken every precaution against deception, sometimes going into the house at eleven or twelve o'clock at night, without being announced, but have always found her the same, and lying in the same position occupied by her for the entire period of her invalidity. The springs of her bedstead are actually worn out with the constant pressure. My brethren in the medical profession at first were inclined to laugh at me, and call me a fool and spiritualist when I told them of the long abstinence and keen mental powers of my interesting patient. But such as have been admitted to see her are convinced. These are Dr. Ormiston, Dr. Elliott and Dr. Hutchison, some of the best talent in the city, who have seen and believed.'"

And then the following account is given of the accident from which the young lady suffered, and to which the remarkable phenomena she is said to exhibit are ascribed:

"The story of Miss Fancher's accident and its melancholy consequences is quite affecting. It is collected from the various statements given by half a dozen friends of the family to the *Herald* reporter. Interwoven with it is a thread of romance, a tale of early love and courtship, of a life embittered by a cruel accident, of patient waiting, and a final release of the suitor from his engagement to marry another.

"Mary's parents live in a sumptuous dwelling on Washington Avenue, Brooklyn, and were reported to be wealthy. Their favorite daughter Mollie, as she was called, was sent to Prof. West's High School in Brooklyn at an early age, and here developed many brilliant qualities of mind and heart, which augured well for her future. At seventeen she was pretty, petite and well cultivated. As a member of the Washington Avenue Baptist Sunday School, she met and learned to love a classmate, named John Taylor. An engagement followed the intimacy of the Sunday School class, and the young people looked forward with buoyant spirits to the bright life so soon to dawn upon them.

"But fate decreed differently. While getting off a Fulton Street car one day in 1864, on her return from school, the young lady slipped and fell backward. Her skirt caught on the step unseen by the conductor, who started the car on its way again. The poor girl was dragged some ten or fifteen yards before her cries were heard and the brake applied. When picked up she was insensible and was carried, suffering intense agony from an injured spine, to her home near by. Forty-eight hours afterward she was seized with a violent spasm which lasted for over two days. Then came a trance, when the sufferer grew cold and rigid, with no evidence of life beyond a warm spot under the left breast, where feeble pulsations of her heart were detected by Dr. Speir. Only this gentleman believed she was alive, and it was due to his constant assertion of the girl's ultimate recovery that Miss Fancher was not buried. Despite the best medical help and the application of restoratives, no change was brought about in the patient's condition until the tenth week, when the strange suspension of life ceased and breath was once more inhaled and breathed forth from her lungs.

"To their dismay the doctors then found that Mollie had lost her sight and the power of deglutition, the latter affliction rendering it impossible for her to swallow food or even articulate by the use of tongue or lip. Previous to her trance a moderate quantity of food had been given her each day; but since then she has not taken a mouthful of life-sustaining food. Spasms and trances alternated with alarming frequency since Miss Fancher was first attacked. First her limbs only became rigid and disturbed at the caprice of her strange malady; but as time passed her whole frame writhed as if in great pain, requiring to be held by main force in order to remain in the bed. She could swallow nothing, and lay utterly helpless until moved."

In the *Sun*, of November 24th, 1878, a fuller account of this young lady was given, mainly however, in regard to her "clairvoyant," or "second-sight" power. Relative to her abstinence from food, I quote the following conversation between the reporter and Dr. Speir.

"'Is it true that she has not partaken of food in all these thirteen years?'

"'No: I cannot say that she has not; I have not been constantly with her for thirteen years; she may have taken food in my absence. Her friends have used every device to make her take nourishment. Food has been forced upon her, and artificial means have been resorted to that it might be carried to her stomach. Nevertheless, the amount in the aggregate must have been very small in all these years.'

"'You have considered the case of such extraordinary importance as to take many physicians to see it?'

"'I have, and it has excited very much of attention. I have letters about it from far and near, and the medical journals have asked for information.'"

And this with Dr. Ormiston:

"Dr. Robert Ormiston, who has been one of Miss Fancher's physicians from the first, who has seen her constantly in all the different conditions of her system, said yesterday that he was convinced that there could be no deception. He could find no motive for it, and he did not believe that she had attempted it. As to her not partaking of food, he had with Dr. Speir made tests that satisfied him that she ate no more than she pretended to, and in the aggregate it had not, in all these years, amounted to more than the amount eaten at a single meal by a healthy man. Dr. Ormiston narrated many curious incidents of the girl's illness, and verified the facts of her physical condition as narrated elsewhere."

In order that no injustice may be done to these gentlemen, I quote the following from the *Sun* of November 26th:

"Dr. R. Fleet Speir, one of Miss Fancher's physicians, smiled last evening when the *Sun* reporter asked him what he thought of Dr. Hammond's opinions on the case. 'I probably have just as high an opinion of Dr. Hammond's opinions as Dr. Hammond has of mine,' he said. 'My opinion on the case of Miss Fancher I have always refused to give to any one. When I first took the case, years ago, I told the family that I would not give them an opinion on it; that I would do what I could with it, and that I hoped to bring about a cure. I do not believe in clairvoyance or second sight, or anything of the kind. I think I stand with the most rigid school on that subject.'

"'But do you think Miss Fancher deceives or endeavors to?'

"The Doctor smiled again. 'Now I do not want you to interview me on that. My theory has along been to do nothing to irritate my patient; I humored her, and have endeavored in that way to get her confidence, to get complete control of her, if possible. In that way I may get her mind diverted, and by and by get her out of bed. I have hoped to see her cured. I do not see what earthly good a scientific investigation would do her. On the contrary, it would harm her. Put a relay of physicians to watch her, and she would undoubtedly do her best to beat them. She would hold out against them, and likely as not die.'

"Dr. Robert Ormiston said that he thought that the Brooklyn physicians knew quite as much about the case as their New York brethren, and that their opinions were of as much weight. 'It has become a most interesting case from a medical standpoint, because during her long illness, she has gone through all the different phases of hysteria that have heretofore been observed in many different cases. I think I am correct in this statement.'"

From all that can be ascertained therefore, it appears that the young lady in question received a severe injury to the spinal cord, in consequence of which she became paralyzed in the lower extremities, in which members contractions also took place. It is probable also that the great sympathetic nerve and brain were involved in the injury.

Confined to her bed, her bodily temperature being low, and passing a good of her time in trances or periods of insensibility, the requirements of the system as regarded food would necessarily be limited. But this is the most that can be said. She *did* breathe, her heart *did* beat, she required *some* bodily heat, and the various other functions of her organism could not have been maintained without the expenditure of matter of some kind. During abstinence from food the body itself is consumed for these purposes, and there being no renovation, no supplies from without, it loses weight with every instant of time until death finally ensues. An emaciated person can withstand this drain less effectually than one who is stout and fat.

Again, it is said that the food taken by Miss Fancher was at once rejected. That it was *all* rejected, is in the highest degree improbable; a portion remained, and this portion, small as it was, did good service when very little was required.

Another point: that Miss Fancher was hysterical admits of no doubt. Hysteria is a disease as much in some cases beyond the control of the patient as inflammation of the brain or any other disease. A proclivity to simulation and deception is just as much a symptom of hysteria as pain is of pleurisy. To say, therefore, that she simulated abstinence and deceived us to the quantity of food she took, is no imputation on her honesty, or questioning her possession of as high a degree of honor and trust, as can be claimed by any one. Other women naturally as moral as she, have under the influence of hysteria perpetrated the grossest deceptions, and they are not unfrequently manifested in the very same way that hers apparently are. Her case is by no means an isolated one; it is not such as has never been seen before; it does not "knock the bottom out of all existing medical theories, and is in a word miraculous," as one of the physicians is reported to have said. On the contrary, similar ones are often met with as we have seen, and the following which I quote from Millingen,[14] is so like it in many respects, that the two might have been formed after a common model, as in fact they were, just as two or more cases of pneumonia follow a well defined type.

"Another wonderful instance of the same kind is that of Janet McLeod, published by Dr. McKenzie. She was at the time thirty-three years of age, unmarried, and from the age of fifteen had had various attacks of epilepsy, which had produced so rigid a lock-jaw that her mouth could rarely be forced open by any contrivance; she had lost very nearly the power of speech and deglutition, and with this all desire to eat or drink. Her lower limbs were contracted towards her body; she was entirely confined to her bed, and had periodical discharges of blood from the lungs, which were chiefly thrown out by the nostrils. During a few intervals of relaxation she was prevailed upon with great difficulty to put a few crumbs of bread comminuted in the hand, into her mouth, together with a little water sucked from her one hand, and, in one or two instances, a little gruel, but even in these attempts almost the whole was rejected. On two occasions also, after a total abstinence of many months, she made signs of wishing to drink some water, which was immediately procured for her. On the first trial the whole seemed to be returned from the mouth, but she was greatly refreshed in having it rubbed upon the throat. On the second occasion she drank off a pint at once, but could not be prevailed upon to drink any more, although her father had now fixed a wedge between her teeth. With these exceptions, however, she seemed to have passed upwards of four years without either liquids or solids of any kind, or even an appearance of swallowing; she lay for the most part like a log of wood, with a pulse scarcely perceptible for feebleness, but distinct and regular. Her countenance was clear and pretty fresh; her features neither disfigured nor sunk; her bosom round and prominent, and her limbs not emaciated. Dr. McKenzie watched her, with occasional visits, for eight or nine years, at the close of which period she seemed to be a little improved."

This account, like that given of Miss Fancher, tells us nothing definite in regard to the fasting abilities of the young woman. It simply, with the other, may be accepted as indicating that hysterical women are able to go for comparatively long periods without food, and that fact we already knew. It will be observed that it is stated that she "*seemed*" to go four years without food or drink.

In regard to Miss Fancher, the evidence is a little conflicting. First we have Dr. Speir reported as saying, in answer to a question as to her having lived fourteen years without food:

"'Yes, she became my patient in 1864. Her case is a most remarkable one.'

"'But has she eaten nothing during all these years?'

"'I can safely say she has not.'"

This in the *Herald*.

But about a month afterward we find the following conversation, reported as taking place between the same physician and another reporter, this time of the *Sun*:

"'Is it true that she has not partaken of food in all these thirteen years?'

"'No, I cannot say that she has not; I have not been constantly with her for thirteen years. She may have taken food in my absence.'"

In which opinion all physiologists will join.

As I have said, hysterical women certainly do exhibit a marked ability to go without both food and drink. I have had patients abstain from sometimes one, sometimes the other, and sometimes both, for periods varying from one day to eleven, and this without much, if any, suffering, for as soon as the suffering came they did not hesitate to signify their desire to break their voluntary fasts. Real suffering is a condition which the hysterical woman avoids with the most assiduous care.

V.

THE PHYSIOLOGY AND PATHOLOGY OF INANITION.

The opinion that food and drink are necessary to life is so generally accepted by mankind, that few venture to dispute the dictum of Virchow relative to Louise Lateau, "Fraud or miracle." But although it is impossible so far as we know for individuals to continue to exist for months and years without the ingestion of nutriment into the system, it is undoubtedly true that under certain circumstances life can be prolonged for days and weeks without any food of any kind going into the organism.

The body is a machine constructed for the purpose of working. The kinds of work which the body of a man or woman does are many. Every act of perception or sensation, is an act of work; so is every thought, every emotion, every volition. The action of the heart or lungs in the circulation and respiration, the evolution of the animal heat, the various functions of secretion and excretion, digestion, motion, speech, etc., are all so many kinds of work. Now as regards work, it is well known that for its due performance force is required, and it is equally well known that for the development of force, matter that can be metamorphosed is necessary. The engine may be perfect, the water may be in the boiler, but unless there be force in the form of heat there will be no steam; and there will be no heat unless there be fuel in a state of combustion.

The human body differs from any other machine in the fact that it uses its fuel in great part indirectly; only in fact after it has been assimilated and converted into tissues of various kinds. Thus when a muscle contracts, it is the muscle itself which is consumed; when a thought is conceived it is the brain which provides the force; when an emotion is experienced, it is again the brain which is decomposed. The body, therefore, lives by the death of its own substance. It is true, some kinds of food such as alcohol, tea and coffee, and perhaps some others do not require to go farther than the blood to be burned, but these are mainly heat-producing, and not tissue-producing substances. But whether matter be consumed directly or indirectly, all bodily force results from its decomposition, and without this destruction of matter the body would be absolutely incapable of a single functional action of any kind whatever, and its temperature like that of the so-called cold-blooded animals would be that of the surrounding medium, the atmosphere.

The quantity of food required by the system varies like the demands of other machines in accordance with the amount of work which is to be performed. A plowman, other things being equal, consumes more than a watchmaker; just as a locomotive burns more fuel than the little engine that runs a sewing machine; the strong able-bodied active man, one who works his brains and muscles up to their full power, eats more than the weak, emaciated and inactive girl, who passes all her time in the recumbent position in bed; and the latter will, other things being equal, endure for a longer period entire abstinence from food. A little food with such a one goes a great way, the demands of the system are at their minimum, and hence a mouthful of bread, or a little tea and toast taken at long intervals, suffices for the supply of all, or a great portion of the waste of the body. With such a person there is not much intense thought, there is little or no muscular action, the pulsations of the heart do not require to be of much force, the respiration is feeble, digestion is at its lowest point, there are no great demands for animal heat, and in fact if the temperature of the atmosphere of the room in which such a person lies, be kept high, the function of calorification may be almost nothing. Still there must be some food taken. The body, can to a certain extent, be used up in supplying the force required for the several functions without the necessity for an immediate restoration of its tissues, but there is a limit to this, beyond which it is certain death to go.

Chossat[15] has determined this point very accurately by many experiments performed upon doves, pigeons, Guinea pigs, rabbits, etc. He found that as a mean result, death ensued when the body lost four-tenths of its original weight. For instance, a body weighing one hundred pounds, could endure the loss of forty pounds without death necessarily following. Five-tenths or one-half appeared to be the extreme loss of weight in inanition which the body could endure without death resulting.

In addition to the loss of weight the temperature fell rapidly, the action of the heart was lessened, the number and depth of the respirations was diminished, and the excretions gradually became smaller in amount.

Experiments such as those of Chossat on the lower animals, cannot of course be instituted on the human subject, nevertheless nature sometimes performs experiments for us which are not without valuable results; and accidents of various kinds, have also given us important data.

On the 19th of March, 1755, twenty-two persons living in the Alpine village of Bergemoletto, in Piedmont, were buried in their houses by an avalanche or whirlwind of snow. The space covered was about two hundred and seventy feet in length, sixty in breadth, and the snow was over forty-two feet in depth. Notwithstanding all the efforts made by the survivors it was impossible to extricate the buried persons till the 18th of April following. All were dead except three women, who, having found some hay, fed a goat with it, and thus obtained from this animal a pint of milk daily, on which they had managed to sustain life for a month.[16]

In Belgium in the year 1683, four colliers were confined in a coal pit for twenty-four days without anything to eat. On the twenty-fifth day they were taken out. In all that time they had lived on nothing but a little water, which flowed from the walls of the prison in which they were immured.[17]

A case is mentioned by Foderé[18] on the authority of M. Chaussier, in which some workmen were taken out alive after having been confined for fourteen days in a cold damp vault. When released at the end of the time mentioned, their pulses were slow and weak, their animal heat greatly reduced, and respiration barely perceptible. Foderé ascribes their long existence without either food or drink, to the fact that the atmosphere of the vault was exceedingly humid, and that the moisture was absorbed into their bodies, taking the place of water ingested into the stomach.

In another case reported by Dr. Straus,[19] a man sixty-five years of age, was extracted alive from a coal mine, in which he had been imprisoned for twenty-three days. During the first ten days he had a little dirty water, but for the last thirteen days nothing whatever. When taken out he was in a condition of great weakness and emaciation and died after three days, notwithstanding all efforts made to preserve his life.

Cases of prolonged abstinence often occur among the insane, who, under the influence of delusions, or in order to destroy their lives refuse all food. Dr. Willan relates the case of a young man, who, through delusions, refused all food but a little orange juice, and who lived for sixty days on this alone.

Of course such persons, if under the observation of a physician, could be fed forcibly, but through the ignorance of friends or relatives it not unfrequently happens that medical aid is not invoked in time, and serious symptoms, or even death itself, may result. The time at which this last termination ensues varies according to the kind of insanity with which the patient is affected. A general paralytic deprived of all food dies sooner than a healthy person. An insane person suffering from acute mania also resists inanition badly, but one the subject of melancholia often endures the total deprivation of aliment for a long time. Esquirol[20] cites the case of a melancholic who did not succumb till after eighteen days of complete abstinence, and Desbarreaux-Bernard another in which life was prolonged for sixty-one days, but in this case a little broth was taken once. Desportes[21] refers to the case of a woman subject to melancholia who continued to exist during two months of abstinence, during which she took nothing into the stomach but a little water.

It would be easy to go on and quote other instances occurring among prisoners, shipwrecked persons, those suffering from diseases which prevented food entering the stomach, others lost in deserts, forests, etc., in which life has been prolonged for considerable periods. Such cases are, however, quite exceptional. An interesting instance occurring under one of these heads may, however, be cited as an example.

M. Lépine[22] reports the case of a young girl nineteen years of age who swallowed a quantity of sulphuric acid. As a consequence a stricture of the œsophagus was produced. Three months after the act, liquids alone passed into the stomach; emaciation was extreme and the countenance pallid. Four months subsequently, that is, seven months after swallowing the acid, the obliteration of the œsophagus was complete, and nothing whatever could be swallowed. The patient lived for sixteen days after all food or drink was prevented reaching the stomach. During the last days of her starvation she complained only of thirst and not of hunger. The prostration was extreme and the temperature greatly lessened. A tendency to sleep was present, and there was a subdued delirium. On the last day of life there was more excitement; the conjunctivæ were red, the pulse thread-like, and the skin cold. It is not stated whether or not attempts were made to feed this patient by injections into the rectum of nutritious substances, or by the use of baths containing such matters in solution. It may, however, safely be taken for granted that efforts of these kinds were made, and if so, the unusually long period during which life was sustained is explained.

In all the cases in which life was extraordinarily prolonged there was either not a total deprivation of food and drink, or there was a state of muscular inaction present particularly favorable to retardation of the destructive changes in the body which abstinence produces. It may be asserted that in ordinary cases absolute deprivation of food and drink cannot be endured by a healthy adult longer than ten days, and death generally ensues before the end of the eighth day. It is said that women sustain abstinence better than men. Young persons and the aged certainly resist with less power than those of the middle period of life. Dante was aware of this fact when he made the children of Ugolino die before their father, the youngest first, the oldest last.

Even though there be a total deprivation of what may strictly be called food, some of the cases already cited show that if water be taken life is preserved for a much longer period than would otherwise be the case. Thus a negro woman, according to Dr. J. W. Francis,[23] believing herself to be bewitched, abstained from food for three weeks, but during this period took two small cups of water, to which a very little wine had been added.

In a case reported by Dr. McNaughton[24] a longer resistance was maintained.

"The subject of this case was a young man, aged twenty-seven, who for three years immediately preceding his death almost constantly kept his room, apparently engaged in meditation, a Bible his only companion. At the latter end of May, 1829, his appetite began to fail; he ate very little, and on the 2d of July he declined eating altogether. For the first six weeks of his fast he went regularly to the well, washed himself, and took a bowl full of water with him into the house. With this he occasionally washed his mouth and drank a little; the quantity taken during the twenty-four hours did not exceed a pint. On one occasion he went three days without taking water, but on the fourth morning he was observed to go to the well and drink copiously and greedily. For the first six weeks he walked out every day, and sometimes spent the greater part of the day in the woods. He retained his strength until a short time before his death. During the first three weeks he emaciated rapidly; afterwards he did not seem to waste so sensibly. Prof. Willoughby visited him a few days before he died. He found the skin very cold, the respiration feeble and slow, but otherwise natural; but the effluvia from the breath, and perhaps the skin, were extremely offensive. During the greater part of the latter week of his life the parents say there was a considerable discharge of foul reddish matter from the lungs. To this perhaps the offensive smell referred to may be chiefly attributed. The pulse was regular, but slow and feeble, and the arteries extremely contracted. The radial artery, for example, could be distinctly felt like a small, hard thread, communicating almost a wiry feel.

"The alvine evacuations were rare; it is believed that he passed several weeks without any, but the secretion of urine seemed more regular. He died after fasting fifty-three days. On dissection the stomach was found loose and flabby. The gall bladder was distended with a dark, muddy-looking bile. The mesentery, stomach and intestines were excessively thin and transparent. There was no fat in the omentum."

In cases of complete abstinence, the phenomena—to several of which attention has already been called—are very striking. The respiration becomes slow until just before death, when, as Chossat observes, there is often a quickening of the respiratory movements. The exhaled breath has a peculiarly sickening and fetid odor. The pulse loses in force and frequency.

The blood becomes reduced in quantity to such an extent sometimes that, as observed by Collard and Martigny,[25] incisions may be made in various parts of the bodies of animals suffering from inanition without there being any hæmorrhage.

The animal temperature falls, according to Chossat, 8° per day until the day of death, when it reaches 14°; and at the moment life departs, the loss suddenly becomes 30°.

All the secretions are diminished in quantity. This is especially shown as regards the saliva and urine. Even open sores cease to secrete pus.

At first there is pain, the seat of which is referred to the stomach, and which pain in the beginning, being simply a feeling of emptiness, rapidly assumes a gnawing or tearing character. But before long this fades away and it does not appear that in the middle and final stages of inanition there is any suffering which can be called a pain, or which can be fixed in any definite part of the body.

The mental faculties are profoundly affected. A high state of delirium supervenes, and there are often hallucinations. These sometimes relate to food, which appears to the sufferer to be spread out before him in the most seducing manner. All nobility of character disappears, and selfishness and brutality govern. Finally the delirium becomes low and muttering, the bodily weakness becomes excessive, walking, or even standing, is impossible, the sufferer loses all sensation, and death ensues.

But probably no part of the subject is of more interest than that which relates to the association of inanition with hysteria. As is well known by physicians, the existence of this latter condition enables many to bear partial, or even complete deprivation of food longer and with less apparent suffering than would be possible with individuals in good health.

That Miss Fancher is subject to hysteria is very evident from a consideration of the clinical history of her case, and hence it is to be expected that she can endure long fasts without much inconvenience. It is just possible that she might, by remaining quietly in bed in a state of partial or complete trance—a hysterical condition in which the waste of the tissues is greatly reduced—exist for a month without either food or drink, and therefore the proposition which I made to her friends contains no exacting condition. But when it is gravely said that "for a period of nearly fourteen years she has lived absolutely without food or nourishment of any kind," we are forced to declare, in the interest of science, that the statement is necessarily absolutely devoid of truth. Subsequent statements, as we have seen, modify this fourteen years' claim very materially, and really leave it in doubt whether there was any abstinence at all.

But I think it may safely be believed that Miss Fancher has indulged in frequent long fasts. Hysteria is very frequently marked, not only by the ability to endure lengthened periods of abstinence, but by the abolition of all desire for food, to such an extent that the sight or even idea of aliment of any kind excites loathing and disgust. M. Lasègue,[26] in a very interesting memoir, has discussed this part of the subject with great precision, and has shown that though such patients take very little food they do take some, and that eventually they experience all the symptoms of inanition. He has never seen death result from the abstinence, for as soon as the condition becomes decidedly unpleasant the patient resumes gradually her normal alimentation.

In a case recently under my care, a young lady twenty-three years of age became hysterical in consequence of domestic troubles, and losing all desire for food, took nothing daily but a single cup of chocolate. She persevered in this restricted diet for twenty-nine days, although during the last eight or ten she gave decided evidences of starvation. She became emaciated, her temperature fell, especially in the extremities, her breath was offensive, her menstruation ceased, and there was such a marked sense of discomfort that she began to crave food, not, as she said, because her appetite had returned, but because she was afraid she would die. Still she resisted till, on the thirtieth day, she begged for a little beef tea, and from that moment her appetite returned to her, and by the end of another week, she was eating her ordinary quantity and variety of food.

Now, in this case, though the amount of nutriment taken daily was small, it was of such a character as to be well able to sustain life. The half pint of chocolate contained milk and sugar, besides the highly nutritious chocolate, with its carbonaceous and nitrogenous matters, and yet a month was the extreme limit of endurance.

That a state of inanition exists in Miss Fancher is not to be doubted. The extreme emaciation, the reduced bodily temperature, the contracted stomach and intestines, the great bodily weakness, all show that she is not sufficiently nourished. In her case there is apparently not only an absence of appetite but a positive disgust for food; and another symptom often present in inanition—vomiting when nutriment is taken into the stomach—appears also to be a prominent feature. It is probable that there is likewise a notable diminution in the amount of urine excreted, as this is a common accompaniment of hysterical manifestations such as hers. In some instances the function appears to be almost entirely arrested, as was the fact in a case described by M. Charcot,[27] and in two which have come under my own observation.

There is nothing remarkable in the admitted fact that Miss Fancher eats very little. We have seen how existence can be kept up on greatly reduced quantities of food, and under circumstances such as those governing her case, for periods which would be impossible in healthy persons. No one yet under any conditions, whether of hysteria or trance or assumed miraculous interference, has, to the satisfaction of competent and disinterested investigators, lived even two months without the ingestion of any food whatever. As to going nearly fourteen years in a state of abstinence—a statement in her behalf which many persons believe to be true—I can only say that all the teachings of science and of experience are against the claim. No one who had the most superficial idea of what knowledge is and how facts can be proven, would for a moment accept such a preposterous story, no matter by whom asserted.

The whole subject is one which is to be examined into and determined like any other matter, and yet, when a proposition is made to investigate by skilled observers the remarkable claim put forward, it is met with abuse and misrepresentation, as if these people thought that all they had to do was to make an assertion of a phenomenon which, according to what we know of nature, is absurd and impossible, to have it at once accepted by those who know, by painful experience, how doubtful all things are till they are proven, and how difficult it is to get satisfactory evidence of the most simple event in physiology or pathology. No one doubts the abstract possibility of a human being living without food, for, bearing in mind the discoveries that are constantly being made, nothing can be regarded as absolutely impossible outside the domain of mathematics. Two and two cannot make six, neither can two distinct bodies occupy the same space at the same time, nor the square of the hypothenuse be otherwise than equal to the sum of the squares of the other two sides of a right-angled triangle.

Our knowledge of natural science is, however, founded on experience. Looking at a bear, for instance, for the first time, and with no knowledge of its habits and capacities we would not be apt to believe that the animal could go into retirement at the beginning of winter and remain till spring in a condition of semi-existence and without food. But experience teaches us that the bear when it begins to hibernate is fat; that during hibernation it is in a perfectly quiescent state; that when it emerges into active life again it is emaciated, and that during the whole period of retirement it has taken nothing into its stomach. We then know by observing that all bears go through the same process, that it is a law of their organism to do so, and that their reduced functional actions are maintained by the consumption of the fat with which in the beginning their bodies were loaded. Even here, then, there is no exception to the law that there is no force without the decomposition of matter. Now, it is just possible that by some hitherto unknown or unrecognized condition of the system a man or woman may obtain the force necessary to carry on life for fourteen years without getting it through food taken into the stomach. But a possibility and a fact are two very different things, and the admitted possibility has not yet been shown to be a fact. It is easier—to use the argument of Hume—for the mind to accept the view that there is deception or error somewhere, than to believe that a woman, contrary to all human experience, should live fourteen years without food. Turtles, we know, will live for months while entirely deprived of nutriment. Many others of the cold-blooded animals will do the same thing. It is their nature to do so, and we have experience of the fact, but it is not the nature of women, so far as we know, and therefore we refuse to accept as true the stories which are told of their powers in this direction. And our knowledge is based not only on our daily experience of the wants of their systems and the examples of starvation which have come to our knowledge, but also upon the fact that in the many cases of alleged long abstinence from food that have been investigated, error or deception has been discovered. Therefore, when it is said that Miss Fancher lives without food, and has so done for fourteen years, we simply say, "give us the proofs." Of course the proofs are not given.

How far Miss Fancher is responsible for the assertions that have been made in regard to her long-continued abstinence I do not know. A tendency to deception is a notable phenomenon of hysteria, and if she has led those about her to accept the view that she has existed without food for years, the circumstance would be in no way remarkable. Other hysterical women have deceived in the same or in still more astonishing ways. Or it may be that the amount of food taken being very small, carelessness or want of exactness has led to the expression that she lived upon "absolutely nothing," just as we hear the words used every day by those who have little or no appetite, but who nevertheless do eat something. Again, a love for the marvellous is so deeply rooted in the average human mind that it willingly, and to a certain extent unconsciously, adds to any statement of a remarkable circumstance, till the latter grows, whilst being repeated, to fabulous dimensions.

But however this may be, whatever the explanation, it is quite certain that if Miss Fancher has lived fourteen years without food, or even fourteen months, or weeks, she is a unique psychological or pathological individual, whose case is worthy of all the consideration which can be given to it, not by superstitious or credulous or ignorant persons, but by those who, trained in the proper methods of scientific research, would know how to get the whole truth of her case, and nothing but the truth. It is to be regretted, therefore, that the proposition contained in the annexed letter (Appendix) was not accepted, and that we are forced to place Miss Fancher's case among the others which have proved to be fallacious, till such time as it may suit her and her friends to allow of such an examination.

FOOTNOTES:

[15] Recherches expérimentales sur l'inanition. Paris, 1843, p. 20.

[16] Universal Magazine, Vol. XXXVI, p. 250.

[17] Abridged Philosophical Transaction, Vol. III, p. 111.

[18] Traité de médecine légale et d'hygiène publique. Paris, 1813. t. II, p. 285.

[19] Medical Gazette, Vol. XVII, p. 389.

[20] Des maladies mentales. Paris, 1838, p. 203.

[21] Du refus de manger chez les aliénés. Thèse de Paris 1864, p.

[22] Nouveau dictionnaire de médecine et de chirurgie pratiques. Paris, 1874. t. XVIII., Art. Inanition, p. 503.

[23] New York Medical and Surgical Journal, Vol. II, p. 31.

[24] Quoted from Trans. of the Albany Institute by Dr. Lee in Copland's Dictionary of Medicine. Vol. I, p. 31.

[25] Recherches expérimentales sur les effets de l'abstinence. *Journal de Physiologie* de Magendie, t. VIII, p. 150.

[26] De l'anorexie hystérique. *Archives générales de médecine,* April 1875.

[27] Leçons sur les maladies du système nerveux, t. I., 2d edition. Paris, 1876, p. 178.

APPENDIX.

The following letter embraces the proposition made to Miss Fancher, to which allusion is made in the text:

To The Editor of the Herald:—

I have read the letter of Professor Henry M. Parkhurst, published in a recent issue of the Herald, relative to the "mind reading" or clairvoyance of Miss Mollie Fancher, of Brooklyn, and it does not satisfy me that the young lady in question possesses any such power. It would have been very easy for her to have opened the envelope without disturbing the seal and to have read the contents. Now, there has been a great deal of talk about Miss Fancher's case. I have received just fifty-seven letters asking me to investigate it, and the press has reiterated the invitation over and over again. I have stated very explicitly that I regard the whole matter as a humbug of the most decided kind, but I have never asserted the impossibility of the young lady's alleged performances. On the contrary, I hold nothing to be absolutely impossible outside the domain of mathematics. But possibilities and realities are very different things, and I certainly will not accept as true any such phenomena as those asserted to have been associated with Miss Fancher unless they are proven.

I have already declared my readiness to investigate Miss Fancher, and, a few days since, in the *Sun*, proposed a test which will be perfectly satisfactory to me and many others who, at present, are in accordance with me in my estimation of this young lady. Permit me now to state it definitely, specifically, and once for all. I will place a certified check for a sum of money exceeding $1,000 inside of a single paper envelope. I will lay the package on a table in the room in which she is. If she chooses she may take it in her hands and place it in contact with any part of her body. I will allow her half an hour to describe the check. If she reads it—number, date, on whom drawn, amount, signature, etc.—accurately, she may have the check as her own property, or I will give the amount expressed in the check, in her name to any charitable institution she may designate, or otherwise dispose of it in accordance with her wishes.

The only conditions I exact are these:—

First—That the experiment be conducted in my presence and in that of two other physicians, members of the New York Neurological Society, whom I will bring with me as witness simply, and who will not interfere in any way with the test.

Second—That the envelope shall at no time pass out of our sight.

If Miss Fancher succeeds in this test I will admit that heretofore in my denunciations of such performances as hers I have been in error, and that there is a force in nature which ought to be investigated. I will pay the money not only without chagrin, but with great satisfaction, and will consider that I have received full value.

If she fails, as I am quite sure she will, I shall not hesitate to continue to denounce her as an imposition in this as well as in her assumed abstinence from food.

A word further in regard to this last matter. I know something about "fasting girls" and their frauds, not excepting the sad case of poor little Sarah Jacob. But I will make this additional proposition:—If Miss Fancher will allow herself to be watched, day and night, for one month, by relays of members of the New York Neurological Society, I will give her $1,000 if at the end of that month she has not in the meantime taken food voluntarily or as a forced measure to save her from dying of starvation, the danger of this last contingency to be judged of by her family physician, Dr. Speir. These offers to remain open for acceptance till twelve o'clock M., December 31st. If not taken up by that time, let us hear no more in support of Miss Fancher's mind reading or clairvoyance, or living for a dozen or more years without food.

WILLIAM A. HAMMOND, M.D.

43 West Fifty-Fourth Street, New York, Dec. 12th, 1878.

Transcriber's Note: Minor typographical errors have been corrected without note, whilst significant amendments have been listed below:

'Nicholas' amended to *Nicolas*
'Aquaintoin' amended to *Aquitaine*
'predominent' amended to *predominant*
'Geraldus Bucoldianus' amended to *Gerardus Bucoldianus*
'fœces' amended to *fæces*
'developes' amended to *develops*
fn. 4, 'Παςατηςήσεων' amended to *Παρατηρήσεων*
fn. 4, added *rararum*: 'medicarum, *rararum*, novarum'
fn. 4, 'monstrasarum' amended to *monstrosarum*
'1567' amended to *1597*
fn. 7, 'chirurgicæ' amended to *chirurgicarum*
, 'Anne Jones' amended to *Ann Jones*
, 'fœcal' amended to *fæcal*
, 'fœces' amended to *fæces*
, 'Cardinal Carrafa' amended to *Cardinal Carafa*
, 'Farenheit' amended to *Fahrenheit*
, fn. 13, 'Rapport Médicale' amended to *Rapport Médical*
, fn. 13, added *de*: 'médecine *de* Belgique'
, 'ecstacy' amended to *ecstasy*
, added *of*: 'direction *of* M. le Curé'

'fecal' amended to *fæcal*
'stigmatisations' amended to *stigmatizations*
'fortell' amended to *foretell*
'marvelous' amended to *marvellous*
'is' amended to *it*: 'that *it* is stated'
'Dr. Spier' amended to *Dr. Speir*
'assimulated' amended to *assimilated*
'alchohol' amended to *alcohol*
'Bergemolletta' amended to *Bergemoletto*
'breath' amended to *breadth*
'Belguim' amended to *Belgium*
fn. 18, 'médicine' amended to *médecine*
'palid' amended to *pallid*
fn. 22, 'Nouvreau' amended to *Nouveau*
fn. 22, 'médicine' amended to *médecine*
'messentery' amended to *mesentery*
'their' amended to *there*
'hemorrhage' amended to *hæmorrhage*
'Chosset' amended to *Chossat*
fn. 26, 'médicine' amended to *médecine*
'her's' amended to *hers*
'injestion' amended to *ingestion*
'Sarah Jacobs' amended to *Sarah Jacob*
'Dr. Spier' amended to *Dr. Speir*

The page reference in fn. 21 (p. 64) was omitted in the original text.

www.ingramcontent.com/pod-product-compliance
Lightning Source LLC
Chambersburg PA
CBHW081126080526
44587CB00021B/3771